MW01290723

Freedom From Fear

What Everyone Ought to Know About Anxiety and Worry

Dr. Robert B. Campbell

Ignited Ministries

4647 Reservoir Rd., Geneseo, NY 14454
www.ignitedministries.org

ignitedministriesinternational@gmail.com

Copyright © 2015 Robert B Campbell

All rights reserved.

ISBN-13: 978-1519272379

ISBN-10: 1519272375

DEDICATION

This book is dedicated to all those who battle fear. May you find freedom as you read about the process that has brought others their freedom.

DISCLAIMER

We are not in competition with nor do not seek to be in conflict with any medical or psychiatric practices, counseling, etc. We do not practice medicine nor do we practice psychology. We are not responsible for anyone's disease or healing. We share insights. All of our work is intended to give insights into healing as we look at possible spiritual roots to disease, sickness and infirmity. We cannot and do not guarantee healing. We have seen incredible results in our work with others. Our insights are not meant to substitute for medical advice or treatment. We do not diagnose or treat disease. We encourage you to seek medical care for your health issues.

All Scriptures are quoted from The New King James Version of the Bible unless stated otherwise.

ACKNOWLEDGMENTS

There are so many that I have drawn from over the years in my search to find healing and wholeness not only for myself but others. My greatest insights have come from my time in the Word of God. Jesus I am thankful!

Isaiah 35:3-10 **Energize** *the limp hands,* **strengthen** *the rubbery knees. 4* **Tell fearful souls**, *"Courage! Take heart! God is here, right here, on his way to put things right And redress all wrongs. He's on his way! He'll save you!" 5* **Blind eyes** *will be opened,* **deaf ears** *unstopped, 6* **Lame men and women** *will leap like deer,* **the voiceless** *break into song.* **Springs of water will burst out in the wilderness, streams flow in the desert**. *7* **Hot sands will become a cool oasis, thirsty ground a splashing fountain**. *Even lowly jackals will have* **water to drink, and barren grasslands flourish richly**. *8 There will be a highway called the Holy Road. No one rude or rebellious is permitted on this road. It's for God's people exclusively — impossible to get lost on this road. Not even fools can get lost on it. 9 No lions on this road, no dangerous wild animals — Nothing and no one dangerous or threatening. Only the redeemed will walk on it. 10 The people God has ransomed will come back on this road.* **They'll sing as they make their way home to Zion, unfading halos of joy encircling their heads, Welcomed home with gifts of joy and gladness as all sorrows and sighs scurry into the night.** *MSG*

Table of Contents

Why a Book on Fear?

Over and over in my interaction with people that have health issues, I inevitably discover that they have some type of fear at work in their lives. That fear can take the form of stress, anxiety, fear, apprehension, worry, tension, etc. The amazing thing to me is that as I study healing and treatment for those maladies and diseases, almost without exception, fear is a major contributor to that sickness or disease. More and more the medical community is making that same discovery. They call it the "mind-body connection" to health. Of course this is not an insight God is unaware of. Rather, He has given us insights all through the Scriptures that link the issues of the heart and what we think to our health. I believe that if you will employ these principles and truths presented in the pages of this book, you will find freedom from fear, stress and anxiety which in turn will release your healing!

Dr. Robert B. Campbell

Fear and the Spirit of Fear

One of the most predominant strongholds in the lives of people everywhere is fear. Everyone experiences it at one time or another. Some battle it every day of their life. Some have grown accustomed to its presence and see it as a normal part of life that must be put up with. Still others see it as a part of their personality therefore nothing can be done about it.

Some fears are not based on reality. There are fears for everything. Fear can come out of nowhere. Whether real or imagined, fear is still a controlling presence in a person's life that needs to be conquered.

Fear and Stress Are Not About Events

Stress is not about events and experiences nearly so much as it is about a person's perception of the circumstances that occur in his or her life. A person's stress level has to do with what a person believes.[i]

What you believe, what you perceive, determines how much stress you have, and the amount of stress determines how tired you feel at the end of the day."[ii]

Is this the way God meant for us to live? NO! You are about to discover how to overcome and dominate fear and the spirit of fear. I have taught hundreds if not thousands how to overcome and dominate fear and the spirit of fear.

How Common is Fear?

According to the National Institute of Mental Health Anxiety Disorders affect about 40 million American adults age 18 years and older (about 18%) in a given year,1 causing them to be filled with fearfulness and uncertainty. Unlike the relatively mild, brief anxiety caused by a stressful event (such as speaking in public or a first date), anxiety disorders last at least 6 months and can get worse if they are not treated. Anxiety disorders commonly occur along with other mental or physical illnesses, including alcohol or substance abuse, which may mask anxiety symptoms or make them worse. In some cases, these other illnesses need to be treated before a person will respond to treatment for the anxiety disorder.[iii]

Here are some recent statistics related to stress and how it is affecting millions in America.

...The sheer stress of living in today's America is driving tens of millions to the point of illness, depression and self-destruction. Consider the following trends:

- *Suicide has surpassed car crashes as the leading cause of injury death for Americans. Even more disturbing, in the world's greatest military, more U.S. soldiers died last year by suicide than in combat;*

- *Fully one-third of the nation's employees suffer chronic debilitating stress, and more than half of all "millennials"*

(18 to 33 year olds) experience a level of stress that keeps them awake at night,including large numbers diagnosed with depression or anxiety disorder.

- *Shocking new research from the federal Centers for Disease Control and Prevention shows that one in five of all high-school-aged children in the United States has been diagnosed with ADHD,and likewise a large new study of New York City residents shows, sadly, that one in five preteens – children aged six to 12 – have been medically diagnosed with either ADHD, anxiety, depression or bipolar disorder;*

- *New research concludes that stress renders people susceptible to serious illness, and a growing number of studies now confirm that chronic stress plays a major role in the progression of cancer,the nation's second-biggest killer. The biggest killer of all, heart disease, which causes one in four deaths in the U.S., is also known to have a huge stress component;*

- *Incredibly, 11 percent of all Americans aged 12 and older are currently taking SSRI antidepressants – those highly controversial, mood-altering psychiatric drugs with the FDA's "suicidality" warning label and alarming correlation with school shooters. Women are especially prone to depression, with a stunning 23 percent of all American women in their 40s*

3

and 50s – almost one in four – now taking antidepressants, according to a major study by the CDC;

- *Add to that the tens of millions of users of all other types of psychiatric drugs, including (just to pick one) the 6.4 million American children between 4 and 17 diagnosed with ADHD and prescribed Ritalin or similar psycho-stimulants. Throw in the 28 percent of American adults with a drinking problem, that's more than 60 million, plus the 22 million using illegal drugs like marijuana, cocaine, heroin, hallucinogens and inhalants, and pretty soon a picture emerges of a nation of drug-takers, with hundreds of millions dependent on one toxic substance or another – legal or illegal – to "help" them deal with the stresses and problems of life.*

By the way, things are no better over the pond – and may be worse, according to one major study that concluded almost 40 percent of Europeans are plagued by mental illness.[iv]

The Most Common Fears

The most common phobias in psychology include irrational fears of spiders, heights phobia, confined spaces, lightning and strangers. Fear of public speaking and fear of flying are also common phobias.[v] Fear almost always relates to future events.

Fear Destroys Our Health

Fear is the major anchor of most illness and disease. It is the root system that feeds and supplies illness and disease with the nutrients they need to flourish. Here is a list of 10 diseases related to fear (stress) that we can actually do something about by getting rid of the fear, stress and anxiety.

10 Health Problems Related to Stress That You Can Fix

The medical community is discovering the link between fear, stress, anxiety and disease. We can continue to deal with the fruits through medication, surgery, etc., or we can go for the root and see genuine healing take place. *What are some of the most significant health problems related to stress? Here's a sampling.*

1. *Heart disease. Researchers have long suspected that the stressed-out, type A personality has a higher risk of high blood pressure and heart problems. We don't know why, exactly. Stress might have a direct effect on the heart and blood vessels. It's also possible that stress is related to other problems -- an increased likelihood of smoking or obesity -- that indirectly increase the heart risks.*
Doctors do know that sudden emotional stress can be a trigger for serious cardiac problems, including heart attacks. People who have chronic heart problems need to avoid acute stress as much as they can.

2.   ***Asthma.*** *Many studies have shown that stress can worsen asthma. Some evidence suggests that a parent's chronic stress might even increase the risk of developing asthma in their children. One study looked at how parental stress affected the asthma rates of young children who were also exposed to air pollution or whose mothers smoked during pregnancy. The kids with stressed out parents had a substantially higher risk of developing asthma.*

3.   ***Obesity.*** *Excess fat in the belly seems to pose greater health risks than fat on the legs or hips -- and unfortunately, that's just where people with high stress seem to store it. "Stress causes higher levels of the hormone cortisol," says Winner, "and that seems to increase the amount of fat that's deposited in the abdomen."*

4.   ***Diabetes.*** *Stress can worsen diabetes in two ways. First, it increases the likelihood of bad behaviors, such as unhealthy eating and excessive drinking. Second, stress seems to raise the glucose levels of people with type 2 diabetes directly.*

5.   ***Headaches.*** *Stress is considered one of the most common triggers for headaches -- not just tension headaches, but migraines as well.*

6.   ***Depression and anxiety.*** *It's probably no surprise that chronic stress is connected with higher rates of depression and anxiety. One survey of recent studies found that people who had stress related to their jobs -- like demanding work with few rewards -- had an 80% higher risk of developing depression within a few years than people with lower stress.*

7.   ***Gastrointestinal problems.*** *Here's one thing that stress doesn't do -- it doesn't cause ulcers. However, it can make them worse. Stress is also a common factor in many other GI conditions, such as chronic heartburn (GERD) and IBS, Winner says.*

8.   ***Alzheimer's disease.*** *One animal study found that stress might worsen Alzheimer's disease, causing its brain lesions to form more quickly. Some researchers speculate that reducing stress has the potential to slow down the progression of the disease.*

9.   ***Accelerated aging.*** *There's actually evidence that stress can affect how you age. One study compared the DNA of mothers who were under high stress -- they were caring for a chronically ill child -- with women who were not. Researchers found that a particular region of the chromosomes showed the effects of accelerated aging. Stress seemed to accelerate aging about 9 to 17 additional years.*

10.   ***Premature death.*** *A study looked at the health effects of stress by studying elderly caregivers looking after their spouses -- people who are naturally under a great deal of stress. It found that caregivers had a 63% higher rate of death than people their age who were not caregivers.*

Still, you might be wondering why. Why would stress make us sick? Why would an emotional feeling wreck havoc on our bodies?

Stress isn't only a feeling. "Stress isn't just in your head," Winner says. It's a built-in physiologic response to a threat. When you're stressed, your body responds. *Your blood vessels constrict. Your blood pressure and pulse rise. You breathe faster. Your bloodstream is flooded with hormones such as cortisol and adrenaline.*

"When you're chronically stressed, those physiologic changes, over time, can lead to health problems."[vi] So the solution is to eliminate the stress, fear and anxiety and you will see these disease vanish!

Definition of Fear

Definition of FEAR Merriam-Webster

1 archaic : frighten

2 archaic : to feel fear in (oneself)

3 to **have a reverential awe of <fear God>**

4 to be afraid of : **expect with alarm** <fear the worst>[vii]

 Fear is a distressing negative emotion induced by a perceived threat. It is a basic survival mechanism occurring in response to a specific stimulus, such as pain or the threat of danger. In short, fear is the ability to recognize danger and flee from it or confront it, also known as the Fight or Flight response. **Worth noting is that fear almost always relates to future events**, *such as worsening of a situation, or continuation of a situation that is unacceptable. Fear could also be an instant reaction to something presently happening.*

Wikipedia (Though I don't look to Wikipedia as an authoritative source it is sometimes useful for simplifying some concepts)[viii]

Quotes on Fear

Fear sees just what man sees. Faith sees what God sees, and acts upon it. Faith creates action, and people of action, like Caleb and Joshua. Unbelief keeps us tied down in a spiritual wilderness – as Israel was for so many years. Without faith, we fear failure and mockery. By faith, we move into God's fullness. ~**REINHARD BONNKE**

Fear is a darkroom where negatives develop. ~**Usman B. Asif**

There is a time to take counsel of your fears, and there is a time to never listen to any fear. ~**George S. Patton**

Many of our fears are tissue-paper-thin, and a single courageous step would carry us clear through them. ~**Brendan Francis**

Fear is faith that it won't work out. ~**Sister Mary Tricky**

To fear is one thing. To let fear grab you by the tail and swing you around is another. ~**Katherine Paterson**

Fear cannot take what you do not give it. ~**Christopher Coan**

He who fears something gives it power over him.
~Moorish Proverb

Feed your faith and your fears will starve to death.
~Author Unknown

What's the Difference Between a Fear and a Phobia?[ix]

The difference between normal fear and a phobia	
Normal fear	**Phobia**
Feeling anxious when flying through turbulence or taking off during a storm	Not going to your best friend's island wedding because you'd have to fly there
Experiencing butterflies when peering down from the top of a skyscraper or climbing a tall ladder	Turning down a great job because it's on the 10th floor of the office building
Getting nervous when you see a pit bull or a Rottweiler	Steering clear of the park because you might see a dog
Feeling a little queasy when getting a shot or when your blood is being drawn	Avoiding necessary medical treatments or doctor's checkups because you're terrified of needles

Fear Is No Respecter of Persons

Louis Pasteur is reported to have had such an irrational fear of dirt and infection he refused to shake hands.

President and Mrs. Benjamin Harrison were so intimidated by the newfangled electricity installed in the White House they didn't dare touch the switches. If there were no servants around to turn off the lights when the Harrisons went to bed, they slept with them on. Jane Goodsell, Not a Good Word About Anybody, Ballantine.[x]

What Causes Phobias?

Some phobias develop when someone has a scary experience with a particular thing or situation. A tiny brain structure called the amygdala (pronounced: uh-mig-duh-luh) keeps track of experiences that trigger strong emotions. Once a certain thing or situation triggers a strong fear reaction, the amygdala warns the person by triggering a fear reaction every time he or she encounters (or even thinks about) that thing or situation.

Someone might develop a bee phobia after being stung during a particularly scary situation. For that person, looking at a photograph of a bee, seeing a bee from a distance, or even walking near flowers where there could be a bee can all trigger the phobia.

Sometimes, though, there may be no single event that causes a particular phobia... People who have had strong childhood fears or anxiety may be more likely to have one or more phobias.

Having a phobia isn't a sign of weakness or immaturity. It's a response the brain has learned in an attempt to protect the person. It's as if the brain's alert system triggers a false alarm, generating intense fear that is out of proportion to the situation. Because the fear signal is so intense, the person is convinced the danger is greater than it actually is.[xi]

Fears As Children

Fear is not something only adults face. It is a common threat to children as well. Common fears among children would include fear of strangers, fear of separation, fear of animals, fear of the dark and fear of thunderstorms.

One summer night during a severe thunderstorm a mother was tucking her small son into bed. She was about to turn the light off when he asked in a trembling voice, "Mommy, will you stay with me all night?" Smiling, the mother gave him a warm, reassuring hug and said tenderly, "I can't dear. I have to sleep in Daddy's room." A long silence followed. At last it was broken by a shaky voice saying, "The big sissy!" **Unknown**.[xii]

As a child, I was afraid when alone in my room. I would imagine an alligator or something under my bed. In order to avoid the alligator I would jump from the bed as far as I could and run out of the room. There was nothing logical about my fear, but it had a grip on me. Fears do not have to make sense.

Media and Fear in Children

By the time the average young person in our culture reaches adulthood, he or she has witnessed more than seventy thousand simulated murders on television." The mind of a child does not differentiate simulated murders from those that are real. The mind perceives danger and responds to danger. We all know that feeling we get while watching a particularly suspenseful or frightening movie. The body experiences a momentary adrenaline response. The same thing can happen if we perceive a wad of lint as being a spider: the adrenaline flows even if the spider is only imaginary. The same is true for a child witnessing potentially deadly events. The stimulation is there-even if the event isn't really there.[xiii]

While I was teaching on fear and sources of fear, someone realized why their children battled fear. They regularly would get their children together on their bed with a bunch of pillows and popcorn and watch scary movies together. They did this because their parents did so with them. They had looked at it as a fun family event. This so-called fun event was releasing fear in the lives of their children.

5-year old Johnny was in the kitchen as his mother made supper. She asked him to go into the pantry and get her a can of tomato soup, but he didn't want to go in alone. "It's dark in there and I'm scared." She asked again, and he persisted. Finally she said, "It's OK-- Jesus will be in there with you." Johnny walked hesitantly to the door and slowly opened it. He peeked inside, saw it was dark, and started to leave when all at once an idea came, and he said: "Jesus, if you're in there, would you hand me that can of tomato soup?"
Charles Allen, Victory in the Valleys.[xiv]

This child had an irrational fear that was

controlling certain areas of his life. Many times adults have these same kinds of irrational fears as well.

Self-Test: Are You Fearful?

Ask yourself these questions to help determine if you have a tendency toward fear and worry.

- Are you afraid of losing your health or wealth or of something bad happening to one you love?
- Do you have trouble sleeping because you are up at night imagining all the things that could go wrong?

- Do you tend to have anxious thoughts about the same thing over and over?

- Do others ever kid you about being a worrywart?

- Do you have a nervous habit like tapping your foot or drumming your fingers?

- Have you ever sought treatment for stress-related symptoms?

- Do you hesitate to make plans because you are worried that things will not turn out well?

- Are your thoughts of the future filled with fear instead of hope?

When we are not trusting in God's care for us, we naturally react to our circumstances by trying to figure out how we can meet our own needs.[xv] That in itself increases the stress level as most of the time we feel limited in what we can do.

A perfect example of someone who had incredible fear is Janez Rus. This man hid for 32 years fearing punishment for his pro-Nazi wartime activity. He was a young shoemaker when he went into hiding at his sisters farmhouse in June of 1945. He was found 32 years later. He said he used to cry when he heard happy voices outside. He didn't even dare go to his own mother's funeral. Throughout those years he did nothing. He never left the house, and could only look down at the village in the valley. He was a victim of his own fears.[xvi]

Can you imagine the life this man lived? Incredible! and yet there are many today living in the prison of fear. Some are in the prison of the fear of rejection, fear of failure, fear of a loss of wealth, fear of a job loss, etc.

What Does The Bible Say About Fear?

> *2 Timothy 1:7 For God has not given us a spirit of **fear**, but of power and of love and of a sound mind. NKJV*

Let's look into the meaning of the word fear as used in this passage.

NT:1167 (fear) state of fear because of a lack of courage or moral strength - 'cowardice, timidity.' fearfullness, [xvii]

Fear Is A Spirit

As you read the passage from 2 Timothy you learn that fear is a spirit. Fear is faith in the wrong direction! Fear neutralizes faith. Fear allows you to be dominated by faithless expectations instead of faith-filled expectations. It is agreement with the wrong kingdom (darkness). Fear is the weapon the enemy uses to steal faith. There was no fear in the garden before sin. There was no stress, no anxiety, no worry. That all came with the fall of mankind and the embracing of a different worldview.

Fear is a demon assigned to bring you into bondage and to restrict your ability to walk in faith. What has God given us? Power and love and a sound mind. Fear produces the opposite. Weakness, insecurity and a "crazy, insane, unreasonable, unsound, unstable" mind.[xviii]

> *1 John 4:18 There is no **fear** in love; but perfect love casts out **fear**, because **fear** involves **torment**. But he who **fears** has not been made perfect in love .NKJV*

Let's look into the meaning of the words fear and torment used in this passage.

*NT:5401 (**fear**: Occurs 47 times in the NT) phobos (fob'-os); from a primary phebomai (to be put in fear); alarm or fright: KJV - be afraid, exceedingly, fear, terror.[xix]*

a state of severe distress, aroused by intense concern

16

for impending pain, danger,[xx]

*NT:2851 (**torment**) has rather the meaning of punishment because of the violation of the eternal law of God. It is equivalent to géenna (G1067), hell, a final punishment about which offenders are warned by our Lord (Mark 9:43- 48). In this sense it does not have the implication of bettering one who endures such punishment.*[xxi]

There is no fear if we are **IN** the love of God and secure **IN** HIS love. There are no phobias, fears, etc. because we are **IN** LOVE. God is LOVE. We can be made perfect **IN** LOVE as we learn who we are and what HE has given to us as HIS sons and daughters. We will explore this in a bit.

> *John 16:33 These things I have spoken to you, that **in** Me you may have **peace**. In the world you will have **tribulation**; but **be of good cheer, I have overcome the world**." NKJV*

Let's look into the meaning of the word IN as used in the passages we just read.

*NT:1722 (**IN**) (A) Particularly with the meaning of in or within as in a ship; in the synagogues, of the believer's union with God; of the mutual union of God and Christ. A fixed position in (place, time or space)*[xxii]

The same word for in is used in the verses below. If you do not know you are IN Christ you will not walk IN Christ but in your own efforts and understanding.

It is almost as if I am inside Christ seeing through His eyes, feeling what He feels, thinking as He thinks, behaving as He behaves! I am IN Him!! I am one with him in heart, mind, and will! He says I am the vine you are the branches. I am fixed in place, in time in space, IN Christ! If I have fear it is because I have stepped out of Christ, out of my place, out of the ship, and out of union with Him. IF I keep His commandments I abide IN His love! If I do not I loose my joy and victory over the enemy and his strategies.

> *John 15:10-11 If you keep My commandments, you will abide in My love, just as I have kept My Father's commandments and abide in His love. 11 "These things I have spoken to you, that My joy may remain in you, and that your joy may be full. NKJV*

His plan is for me to have joy to the full. If I am walking in fear, stress and anxiety there is no abundance of joy!

> *2 Cor 5:17 Therefore, if anyone is **in** Christ, he is a new creation; old things have passed away; behold, all things have become new. NKJV*

To remain in Christ means I take care of any sin issues as they come up. If I sin by not keeping His commandments I repent, ask for His forgiveness and my sin is gone and I am back IN right standing with

Him.

> *John 15:3-8 Abide* (one with him in heart, mind, and will[xxiii]) ***in** Me, and I **in** you. **As the branch cannot bear fruit of itself, unless it abides in the vine, neither can you, unless you abide in Me.*** *5 "I am the vine, you* are *the branches.* **He who abides in Me, and I in him, bears much fruit**; *for* **without Me you can do nothing**. *6 If anyone does not abide in Me, he is cast out as a branch and is withered; and they gather them and throw them into the fire, and they are burned.* **(goes along with fear involves torment because I am not one with Him in heart, mind, and will)** *7 If you abide in Me, and My words abide in you, you will* ask what you desire, and it shall be done for you. 8 By this My Father is glorified, that you bear much fruit; so you will be My disciples. NKJV*

As we abide IN Him we bear much fruit! If I do not abide IN Him I wither away and become *unproductive and unfruitful. Why? Because I am not one with Him in heart, mind and will and I am trying to do it in my own strength. Now let's get back to John 16:33*

> *John 16:33 These things I have spoken to you, that **in** Me you may have **peace**. In the world you will have **tribulation**; but **be of good**

> **cheer, I have overcome (conquered and gotten the victory over) the world."** *NKJV*

When we are fearful, full of stress and anxiety, we do not have peace. IN Jesus we have peace but IN the world we will have tribulation or trouble. It is a choice we make. We will look at peace and its meaning after we look at life without it which is tribulation as stated in John 16:33.

Here's the definition of tribulation.

*NT:2347 (**Tribulation**), Trouble : pressure, distress (to afflict with great pain, anxiety, or sorrow; trouble; worry; bother. To subject to pressure, stress, or strain; embarrass or exhaust by strain: to be distressed by excessive work. Also crush, press, compress, squeeze, which is from thlao (n. f.), to break. Tribulation, trouble, affliction.*

(I) In a figurative manner, pressure from evils, affliction, distress like of a woman in travail[xxiv]

Let me explore with you a different take on this verse. There is an additional meaning within the verse. The same definition of IN is used for both In Christ and IN the world. If I am IN the world, I am one with the world's ways of doing things in heart, mind, and will. If I do that I will be ***afflicted with great pain, anxiety, or sorrow. I will be troubled, worried and bothered. I will be subject to pressure, stress, or strain and squeezed and compressed by the stress. I will be***

embarrassed or exhausted by strain and distressed by excessive work. Sounds like the abundant life doesn't it?

Jesus says in Matthew 11:30 that His yoke is easy and His burden light! So if I remain or abide in Him (one with him in heart, mind, and will[xxv]) I too will overcome. It is not by my might nor my power but by His Spirit at work in me![xxvi] I am not saying we won't have any trouble, but Jesus reminds us that He overcame. Not only do I overcome but I have HIS peace in the midst of my tribulation and trouble. Let's look at the meaning of the word peace used in this passage as well as a Messianic prophecy about Jesus.

> Isaiah 9:7 Of the increase of His government and **peace** There will be no end...NKJV

Let's look into the meaning of Peace from this Old Testament passage as it mirrors the New Testament meaning of peace.

OT7965 (PEACE) salom; or shalom; from 7999; **safe,** *i. e. (figuratively)* **well, happy,** *friendly; also (abstractly)* **welfare,** *i. e.* **health, prosperity, peace:— (good) health, prosper (- ity,- ous), rest, safe (- ty),** *soundness, welfare, peace completeness (in number) safety, soundness (in body) welfare, health, prosperity peace, quiet, tranquillity, contentment peace, friendship of human relationships with God especially in covenant relationship[xxvii] Now let's look at the meaning of peace* *in the gospel of John.*

> *John 14:27* **Peace** *I leave with you,* **My peace** *I give to you; not as the world gives do I give to you.* **Let not your heart be troubled, neither let it be afraid.** *NKJV*

Here's the definition:

NT 1515 (Peace) meaning health, welfare, prosperity, every kind of good.[xxviii]

This sounds like the abundant life He promised! This is all ours as His gift to us if we are one with him in heart, mind, and will. What if this is not what you are experiencing? This can be yours! We will look at a plan of action to obtain this peace after we explore some of the ways fear has gotten into our lives.

Entry Points
If we can it is helpful to understand the root of your fear. When did it begin? Was there an event? Was there a conflict?

Some have learned fear from others or inherited through their family tree spirits of fear. In some families everyone has the same fear, it is a learned behavior. It has been passed from generation to generation. Some families have been plagued with disease and have in common a fear of that disease. Their expectation and what they say about the disease is actually a type of faith that something bad will come about and it does. Fear is almost as powerful as faith.

Fear is faith in the wrong direction.

Some can obtain a fear through a tragic event or accident. Some fears have come through media either in our childhood or as a teen or adult. There are many ways fear can enter a person's life.

My wife, Kathy, was in a head-on automobile accident a number of years ago. She was not in the wrong, someone turned into her lane and crashed head-on into her vehicle. Fortunately they both survived with some minor injuries. Because that accident was on a road we travelled often, we would have to drive by that location on almost a daily basis. Every time we passed that location, fear would grip her. Her fear was induced by an accident. It didn't matter that she was not at fault, fear gripped her none the less. We can have fears that come as a result of what someone else has done. We still need to overcome those fears.

Some Characteristics of Fear
Fear Is Faith In The Wrong Direction ~ We Need Biblical Faith

> *Job 3:25 For the thing I greatly feared has come upon me, And what I dreaded has happened to me. NKJV*

Job had great faith in the wrong direction (fear) concerning his children. We need Biblical faith in the right direction!

Faith accesses the impossible! Without faith it is impossible to please God.

> *Heb 11:6 But without faith it is impossible to please Him, for he who comes to God must believe that He is, and that He is a rewarder of those who diligently seek Him. NKJV*

Fear is the strategy of the enemy to eliminate your faith in God and your future. Fear and faith both have expectations of the future. Fear and Faith both demand that you believe something that has not yet happened! Whatever we meditate on we give power to.

Fear Is Contagious

Fear is contagious, look at the 10 spies who gave an evil report.[xxix] They said we are like grasshoppers in their sight. That report neutralized about 1.2 million people and kept them from their promised land. Those spies also died of the plague.

Are there fears robbing you of your future? Are you hanging out with people that are filled with fear? Be the agent of change! Start speaking faith!

Fear Is Sin Because It Is An Ungodly Belief

> *Rom 14:23...for whatever is not from faith is sin.* NKJV*

Fear takes many forms such as anxiety, panic attacks, worry, stress, being nervous, apprehension, phobias, etc.

"By definition, phobias are IRRATIONAL, meaning that they interfere with one's everyday life or daily routine. For example, if your fear of high places prevents you from crossing necessary bridges to get to work, that fear is irrational. If your fears keep you from enjoying life or even preoccupy your thinking so that you are unable to work, or sleep, or do the things you wish to do, then it becomes irrational." xxx

> *Matthew 6:34 Therefore do not worry about tomorrow, for tomorrow will worry about its own things. Sufficient for the day is its own trouble. NKJV*

Fear is a Lack of Trust in God and a Lack of Peace

Fear accuses God. We are not able to trust God. If we trust in God we have peace.

False

Evidence

Appearing

Real

It's a façade! It is the enemy asking "Hath God said?" Jesus has given us His Peace! His Health, Welfare, Prosperity and every kind of good! Fear cannot posses that.

> *John 14:27* **Peace** *(health, welfare, prosperity, every kind of good) I leave with you, My* **peace** *(health, welfare, prosperity, every kind of good) I give to you; not as the world gives do I give to you. Let not your heart be troubled, neither let it be afraid. NKJV*

> *John 16:33 These things I have spoken to you, that in Me you may have* **peace**. *(health, welfare, prosperity, every kind of good) In the world you will* have tribulation; but be of good cheer, I have overcome the world." NKJV*

Fear can open the door to sickness and calamity.

> *Job 3:25 For the thing I* ***greatly feared*** *has come upon me, and what I dreaded has happened to me. (NKJ)*

Fear Separates Us From God and Brings Torment

Fear destroys lives. Fear seeks to govern our actions. Fear eliminates our ability to live in love. The way to conquer fear is through perfect love.

> *1 John 4:18 There is no fear in love; but perfect love casts out fear, because fear involves torment (torment or punishment). But he who fears has not been made perfect in love. NKJV*

26

How Fear Works

When we sense danger, the brain reacts instantly, sending signals that activate the nervous system. This causes physical responses, such as a faster heartbeat, rapid breathing, and an increase in blood pressure. Blood pumps to muscle groups to prepare the body for physical action (such as running or fighting). Skin sweats to keep the body cool. Some people might notice sensations in the stomach, head, chest, legs, or hands. These physical sensations of fear can be mild or strong.

This response is known as "fight or flight" because that is exactly what the body is preparing itself to do: fight off the danger or run fast to get away. The body stays in this state of fight-flight until the brain receives an "all clear" message and turns off the response.

Sometimes fear is triggered by something that is startling or unexpected (like a loud noise), even if it's not actually dangerous. That's because the fear reaction is activated instantly — a few seconds faster than the thinking part of the brain can process or evaluate what's happening. As soon as the brain gets enough information to realize there's no danger ("Oh, it's just a balloon bursting — whew!"), it turns off the fear reaction. All this can happen in seconds. [xxxi]

Fear Is Sometimes Useful; Fight Or Flight

Several bodily changes occur as a reaction to a fearful event. During fear, hormones that prepare us

27

to adapt to stress are released in a chain reaction, first from the brain, which trigger in turn the release of stress hormones from the adrenal glands. Our heart rate increases, blood is redirected to body parts associated with fight or flight, and extra sugar is made available in the bloodstream via the liver.

Unresolved fear may convert to anxiety as we begin to grow accustomed to a threat. When we're anxious, the same physical changes that accompany fear occur at lower levels, with harmful effects on our body. Sustained increased heart output and constriction of blood vessels to rechannel blood to certain organs can contribute to the development of high blood pressure and cardiovascular disease. Altered sugar metabolism can worsen diabetes. The tendency for digestive activity to increase in times of stress can exacerbate underlying gastric ulcers.

Worry and anxiety involve recycling the same fear, repeatedly examining the outcomes and evaluating interventions. We sometimes use this activity to justify worry, assuming that repeated scrutiny will result in knowing what to do if worse comes to worst, but this continual rehearsal of negative events in search of solutions may not benefit us should danger actually arise. The two thought processes, worry and planning, center in different parts of the brain. On magnetic resonance imaging, those who worry show activity in the emotional part of the brain, whereas those who plan show activity in the opposite hemisphere, the so-called logical half of the brain. This may mean that, from the standpoint of providing a good solution in the face of danger, worry is not the best strategy. Worry does not determine the best solution and move on to the next problem. It prevents us from detecting and dealing with new problems in a timely and effective way.

Physical symptoms of anxiety may include any of these: shortness of breath, sigh breathing, dry mouth, inability to swallow, trembling, weakness, incessant crying, circular or obsessive thoughts, inability to concentrate, paralytic or manic movements, insomnia, headache, recurrent nightmares, or extreme fatigue.

The effect of stress on the immune system

The stress hormones released by the adrenals during episodes of fear and anxiety also affect white blood cells, the infection-fighting army within our blood. Initially, the surge of brain and adrenal hormones that accompanies stress causes an increase in circulating white blood cells. When cortisol remains high, however, white blood cell numbers are reduced. As stress, anxiety, or depression continue unabated over weeks or months, output of the adrenal hormone cortisol is consistently high and white blood cell numbers remain reduced. [xxxii]

If we continually fear our immune system degenerates and we get weaker and weaker and our health goes downhill. Because fear weakens our immune system, we will equip you on how to strengthen your immune system as we move into ministry.

Cortisol, Stress, ANS, and Anabolic Hormones

Chronic stress, whether emotional or physical, and sympathetic predominance of your nervous system decreases anabolic hormones and anabolic processes and increases cortisol, the most potent anabolic hormone in your body.

Low cortisol allows your body to repair and regenerate itself while you're asleep. If cortisol remains high, you may be able to sleep, but your body doesn't recharge or rebuild. If that pattern continues, things will eventually start to break down.

When the body is able to rebuild during sleep, cortisol will be high upon waking. You will feel recharged and ready to take on the world. If you wake up tired, a low morning cortisol probably has you dragging out of bed.

Under stress, cortisol levels can run very high. Abnormal circadian rhythm normally will not develop until stress is prolonged—usually over years—but it can also occur in just a few months, especially if it is severe and constant.

When the cortisol rhythm stays out of balance, more serious problems can appear, such as arthritis, allergies, asthma, colitis, ulcers, recurrent and prolonged infections, auto-immune diseases, and degeneration of the nervous system.[1]

I have included a chart below that lists the effects of chronically high cortisol.[2]

Effects of Chronically High Cortisol	
System	Effect
Production of Energy	Blood sugar levels and the ability of your cells to make energy are compromised. Insulin resistance results in excess body fat, diabetes, and heart disease.
Sleep	The rapid eye movement stage (REM) of the sleep cycle is interrupted by high cortisol values at night. Since REM is the most regenerative stage of sleep, fatigue, depression, and lack of mental acuity can result.
Brain	Damage to neurons and receptors in your brain. This probably accounts for the problems with depression, learning, and memory observed in people who are chronically stressed.
Muscle and Connective Tissues (Tendons, ligaments, and joints)	Reduced tissue repair, coupled with an increased rate of tissue breakdown (a normal part of body metabolism), leads to an increased risk for muscle and joint injury. The lowered rate of repair and increased breakdown prevents normal repair of injuries, even everyday wear-and-tear, and leads to chronic injuries and chronic pain.
Bone	If the night cortisol is elevated, your bones do not rebuild during sleep and you are more prone to osteoporosis.
Immune System	Decreased production of white blood cells; decreased immune response in the linings of the lungs, throat, kidneys, bladder, and intestinal tract. Lowered resistance to infection and increased risk for allergies.
Skin Regeneration	Thin, dry (even crepe-paper-like) skin. Human skin regenerates mostly during the night while you're asleep. Moist, resilient skin is a sign of healthy cortisol rhythm.
Thyroid Function	High cortisol levels inhibit thyroid hormone levels and result in fatigue, low body temperature, and weight gain.
Pituitary Gland	Low pituitary hormone levels inhibit thyroid, male and female, and growth hormone levels.
Liver	Abnormal cortisol levels stress liver detoxification pathways.
Intestines	Abnormal cortisol levels weaken the intestinal wall, resulting in ulcers, colitis, Crohn's Disease, Irritable Bowel Syndrome, and abnormal gut flora.

---

[1] http://www.theelementsofhealth.com/resources/articles/articles-stress/the_autonomic_nervous_syste.pdf
[2] http://www.theelementsofhealth.com/resources/articles/articles-stress/the_autonomic_nervous_syste.pdf

How Do We Overcome Fear?

We Must Deal With Fear (stress & anxiety) and The Spirit of Fear.

1. **First of all you need to Recognize** whether or not you have any **Fear** (stress and anxiety) as you can open yourself to **Spirits of Fear** operating in your life. These can be passed down generationally in a family as a familiar spirit. We may see it as "that's just the way my family is." That may be true, but you don't have to continue believing that mindset any longer.

> *Psalms 51:6 Behold, You desire truth in the inward parts, And in the hidden part You will make me to know wisdom. NKJV*

2. Take **Responsibility** for your sin. After repenting of any known sin and asking for forgiveness and making restitution where necessary, genuine guilt is eliminated. Now you need to move on to the remaining roots. Agreeing with **Fear** is sin because it is an ungodly belief and a lack of trust of God. Don't blame others. Again, if you have legitimate guilt, repent and ask forgiveness for the sin causing the guilt. If you need to make something right with someone, do so.

3. **Repent** and ask for forgiveness for any known sin. If you have agreed with **Fear,** repent and ask God to forgive you. Ask God to forgive you for not trusting Him and for believing that your issues were beyond His reach, control, care or forgiveness. Ask for

forgiveness from Him for believing He was not out for your good.

4. **Renounce (come out of agreement with)** involvement with **Fear** (stress and anxiety) and the **<u>Spirit of Fear</u>** and command it to leave. State you want nothing to do with **<u>Fear</u>** and the **<u>Spirit of Fear</u>** and command it to leave in Jesus' name.

5. **Resist** the sin of **<u>Fear</u>** and all the enemy's strategies. He will attempt to get you to again agree with **<u>Fear</u>**. This is not a one-time battle over your thought life, but an on-going battle until you see victory! Flee from evil temptation, but pursue righteousness, faith, love and peace.[3]

6. **Reign** over your thought life. Don't allow these sins and ungodly beliefs to dominate your thought life any longer. Adopt a correct view of God. You need to see how willing and capable God is to keep all His promises to you. You also need to revise any false beliefs you have by examining what God says in His Word. Resist worldly values and beliefs contrary to the Word of God. We will provide Scriptures on specific topics at the end of this book. You are the one who takes every thought captive to the obedience of Christ. Believe God and trust His Word!

7. **Reestablish** your authority according to Luke 10:19 and 2 Timothy 1:7. You have authority over all the power of the enemy!

---

[3] 2 Timothy 2:22 NKJV

Remember that the **Spirit of Fear** come as a result of agreement with their kingdom values of fear.

8. **Rest** in who God is. *God with us! A very present help in time of trouble.⁴ Believe His promises! It is God who works in you both to will and to do of His good pleasure. Philippians 2:13*

9. Let the peace of God **Rule** and Reign in your heart by the Holy Spirit. Don't go back to worry and fear, but receive His peace on purpose!

10. **Speak** to **any health issues**. **Command** them to go and your body to be healed in Jesus' name. Command your immune system to come into balance and function properly in Jesus' name. Command the serotonin levels to be restored to normal in Jesus' name. Command the arteries and blood vessels to function properly in Jesus' name. Command all pain to go in Jesus' name. Command all generational curses to be broken and command the **spirit of infirmity** to leave in Jesus' name.

11. Be committed to **Rescuing** others by sharing these truths. This is not about trying to control others, but helping to empower them if they are open to it. The Scripture says ***Gently***!

---

⁴ Psalms 46:1 NKJV

> *2 Timothy 2:25-26 Gently instruct those who oppose the truth. Perhaps God will change those people's hearts, and they will learn the truth. 26 Then they will come to their senses and escape from the devil's trap. For they have been held captive by him to do whatever he wants. NLT*

> *Luke 10:19 Behold, I give you the authority to trample on serpents and scorpions, and over all the power of the enemy, and nothing shall by any means hurt you. NKJV*

I love the way it is worded in the Amplified Bible.

> *Luke 10:19 Behold! I have given you authority and power to trample upon serpents and scorpions, and [physical and mental strength and ability] over all the power that the enemy [possesses]; and nothing shall in any way harm you. AMP*

Luke 10:19 is your foundational Scripture. Memorize it!

Prayer
(It is important to remember this needs to be done out loud as the enemy does not know our thoughts. Our authority is expressed verbally. Jesus said "If you say to the mountain" Mark 11:23. These are not just words to be spoken,

but they must also be mixed with faith and a confidence that God's word is true!)

Lord, forgive me for my sin. I repent of all known sin now. (List them to God) Forgive and cleanse me now. Forgive me for agreeing with **Fear and Anxiety**. I acknowledge that **Fear and Anxiety** is sin. I repent and turn away from **Fear and Anxiety** and the **Spirit of Fear** now. I also ask that You forgive me for not trusting You Father. I know my lack of trusting You has grieved You. Forgive me. Wash me clean. Give me Your strength and ability to live free of **Fear and Anxiety** in Jesus' name. I receive that strength and ability now. Where I have sinned against others, I will ask for their forgiveness and make restitution. I renounce all involvement with **Fear and Anxiety** and the **Spirit of Fear**. **Fear and Anxiety** and the **Spirit of Fear**, I want nothing to do with you any longer. I have authority over all of your power as I have been given that authority over you in Jesus' name according to Luke 10:19. I exercise that authority over you now. You have no legal right to be here as I have repented of agreement with you and so I command you to go now in Jesus' name. I break every generational curse in my life now in Jesus' name.

I now choose to resist all **Fear and Anxiety** and the **Spirit of Fear** in Jesus' name from this time forth. I take authority over all thoughts to the obedience of Christ Jesus. **Fear and Anxiety** will no longer dominate my thought life. God's Word will dominate my thought life from this time forth in Jesus' name. Thank You, Lord, that you are with me. Thank you for Your forgiveness and grace. Thank You for your peace. I receive Your **peace** even now. *(health, welfare, prosperity and every kind of good.)* Jesus, I receive Your health, Your welfare, Your prosperity and every kind of good in Your name now!

I now take authority over _list any disease or malady here_. _list any disease or malady here_ go in Jesus' name. Spirit of infirmity go in Jesus' name! Serotonin levels come back to normal in Jesus' name. Arteries function properly in Jesus' name. Immune system be strengthened and made whole and function properly in Jesus' name! Hormones come into balance in Jesus' name! I command all pain and disease to go now in Jesus' name! Thank You, Lord, that You have forgiven me all my iniquities and You have healed all my diseases. Thank You for my healing now in Jesus' name.

> *Psalms 103:1-5 Bless the Lord, O my soul; And all that is within me, bless His holy name! 2 Bless the Lord, O my soul, And forget not all His benefits: 3 Who forgives all your iniquities, Who heals all your diseases, 4 Who redeems your life from destruction, Who crowns you with lovingkindness and tender mercies, 5 Who satisfies your mouth with good things, So that your youth is renewed like the eagle's. NKJV*

My Prayer For You

Father, I thank you for releasing Your healing grace to this child that You love in Jesus' name. According to Luke 10:19, I take authority over all afflicting and hindering spirits in the name of Jesus and command them to loose their hold and go now in Jesus' name. I command the spirits of Fear and Infirmity to loose their hold and go now in Jesus' name! I take authority over every generational spirit and curse and command them to go in Jesus' name. I command all pain to go now in Jesus' name! Fear go! I command all organs to function properly and all hormones to come into balance now in Jesus' name. I speak a word of restoration over all damage in this body and for healing virtue to flow now in Jesus' name. I speak to the immune system and command it to be healed and restored now in Jesus' name. Healing virtue and peace come now in Jesus' name I pray, amen.

Your Daily Declaration (Spoken out loud based on *Job 22:28 "You will also decree a thing, and it will be established for you; And light will shine on your ways. NASB)*

I am accepted in the beloved. I am loved and cared for by God and I am His workmanship. I have authority over all the power of the enemy and nothing shall by any means hurt me. No weapon formed against me shall prosper in Jesus' name. All fear has gone and I have power, love and a sound mind. I am prospering and enjoying good health even as my soul prospers. My serotonin levels are normal and my immune system is functioning properly in Jesus' name. My organs are functioning properly and my hormones are in balance in Jesus' name. By Jesus stripes I am healed. I receive His strength and restoration into my life and body now. My body is being made new!

The following are adapted from the "Steps To Freedom In Christ" by Neil Anderson.

To maintain freedom commit to the following;

1. **Seek legitimate Christian fellowship** where you can walk in the light and speak the truth in love, where you will be supported in walking out your healing and wholeness.

2. **Renew** your mind by washing it with the Word of God. Study your Bible daily. Memorize key verses. This is how our minds are renewed.

> *Ephesians 5:26 that He might sanctify and cleanse her (the Church) with the washing of water by the word, NKJV*

3. **Realize** who you are in Christ. Christ in you does not fear or worry!

> *Galatians 2:20 I have been crucified with Christ [in Him I have shared His crucifixion]; it is no longer I who live, but Christ (the Messiah) lives in me; and the life I now live in the body I live by faith in (by adherence to and reliance on and complete trust in) the Son of God, Who loved me and gave Himself up for me. AMP*

4. **Reign** over your thought life. Take every thought captive to the obedience of Christ. Assume responsibility for your thought life, reject the lie, choose the truth and stand firm in your position in Christ. Do this daily! Review teachings in this book to remind yourself of the truth in order to walk out your healing and wholeness. Don't drift away! It is very easy to get lazy in your thoughts and revert back to old habit patterns of thinking. Share your struggles openly with a trusted friend. You need at least one friend who will stand with you. Take Every Thought Captive! If this is a struggle for you quote Scriptures out loud. Try thinking of something negative or full of stress while quoting a Scripture out loud, you can't do it!

> *2 Corinthians 10:5 [Inasmuch as we] refute arguments and theories and reasonings and every proud and lofty thing that sets itself up against the [true] knowledge of God; and we lead every thought and purpose away captive into the obedience of Christ (the Messiah, the Anointed One), AMP*

5. **Rest** in who God is. God with you!

> *1 John 4:18 There is no fear in love; but perfect love casts out fear, because fear involves torment. But he who fears has not been made perfect in love. NKJV*

> *Matthew 1:23 "Behold, the virgin shall be with child, and bear a Son, and they shall call His name Immanuel,"* which is translated, "God with us." NKJV*

> *Philippians 4:13 I can do all things through Christ* who strengthens me. NKJV*

6. **Resist** fear and worry. In order for the devil to flee, we need to resist. Nothing comes without warfare. He will try and come back, but you must resist him.

> *James 4:7-8 Therefore submit to God. Resist the devil and he will flee from you. 8 Draw near to God and He will draw near to you. Cleanse your hands, you sinners; and purify your hearts, you double-minded. NKJV*

7. Let the peace of God **Rule** and Reign in your heart by the Holy Spirit. Invite that peace to come now. Remember, the word peace means health, welfare, prosperity and every kind of good!

Colossians 3:15 And let the peace (soul harmony which comes) from Christ rule (act as umpire continually) in your hearts [deciding and settling with finality all questions that arise in your minds, in that peaceful state] to which as [members of Christ's] one body you were also called [to live]. And be thankful (appreciative), [giving praise to God always]. AMP **Peace=Health, welfare, prosperity and every kind of good!**

Romans 15:13 Now may the God of hope fill you with all joy and peace in believing, that you may abound in hope by the power of the Holy Spirit. NKJV Peace=Health, welfare, prosperity and every kind of good!

8. **Renounce** involvement with **Fear and Anxiety** and the **Spirit of Fear** if you stumble. In the book of Acts there were those who were involved in magic (a forbidden practice) and as a sign of repentance they brought all their books on magic and they burned (renounced) those books publicly, so we renounce all involvement with **Fear and Anxiety** and the **Spirit of Fear**.

9. **Don't expect another person to fight your battle for you.** Others can help, but they can't think, pray, read the Bible or choose the truth for you.

Key Scriptures For Victory

Meditate on and apply these verses to your life. If you need to repent in an area, do so and take up your God given authority over all **Fear (stress & anxiety), Anger (possible fits of rage), Rejection, Bitterness, Self-Bitterness, Self-Hatred, Self-Rejection and Condemnation Self-Hatred, Self-Rejection, Condemnation, Fear, Worry and Stress**!

Remember - if it's the truth that sets you free, it's a lie that holds you captive. I don't have the right to pick and choose which thoughts i take captive!

> *John 8:32 and you will know the truth, and the truth will set you free." ESV*

> *2 Timothy 3:16 All Scripture is given by inspiration of God, and is profitable for doctrine, for reproof, for correction, for instruction in righteousness, NKJV*

The challenge with thought is determining its origin. You can have a thought, be convinced it is your own, and follow its influence and direction. You can believe a thought is a great idea, part of your personality, or discernment. You can believe all of those things and you can be walking into the trap of the enemy. We are dealing with a very intelligent being who was able to convince a third of the angels that God was unjust. This was in a perfect, sinless environment. He appealed to their pride by promising something they didn't have. He did the same with Adam and Eve. Pride was his own snare as well. Pride is almost always at the center of wrong or caustic thinking. The challenge is to recognize the origin of our thought. Once we recognize caustic thinking, we displace it with the truth of God's word and refuse to go back into the same thinking patterns. We take every thought captive to obey Christ!

> *2 Corinthians 10:5 We destroy arguments and every lofty opinion raised against the knowledge of God, and take every thought captive to obey Christ, ESV*

God's Faithfulness

God cares for me ~

> *Deuteronomy 7:9 "Therefore know that the Lord your God, He is God, the faithful God who keeps covenant and mercy for a thousand generations with those who love Him and keep His commandments; NKJV*

God is faithful and compassionate ~

> *Lamentations 3:22-23 Through the Lord 's mercies we are not consumed, Because His compassions fail not. 23 They are new every morning; Great is Your faithfulness. NKJV*

God comforts me in my darkest times ~

> *Job 35:10 But no one says, 'Where is God my Maker, Who gives songs in the night, NKJV*

God watches over me ~

> *Psalms 12:5 "For the oppression of the poor, for the sighing of the needy, Now I will arise," says the Lord; "I will set him in the safety for which he yearns." NKJV*

God comforts me ~

> *Isaiah 40:9-11 O Zion, You who bring good tidings, Get up into the high mountain; O Jerusalem, You who bring good tidings, Lift up your voice with strength, Lift it up, be not afraid; Say to the cities of Judah, "Behold your God!" 10 Behold, the Lord God shall come with a strong hand, And His arm shall rule for Him; Behold, His reward is with Him, And His work before Him. 11 He will feed His flock like a shepherd; He will gather the lambs with His arm, And carry them in His bosom, And gently lead those who are with young. NKJV*

God promises to comfort me when I mourn ~

> *Matthew 5:4 Blessed are those who mourn, For they shall be comforted. NKJV*

God's Holy Spirit is my Comforter ~

> *John 14:16 And I will pray the Father, and He will give you another Helper, that He may abide with you forever — NKJV*

God gives power to me ~

> *Isaiah 40:29 He gives power to the weak, And to those who have no might He increases strength. NKJV*

God is my refuge and fortress ~

> *Psalms 91 He who dwells in the secret place of the Most High Shall abide under the shadow of the Almighty. 2 I will say of the Lord , "He is my refuge and my fortress; My God, in Him I will trust." 3 Surely He shall deliver you from the snare of the fowler And from the perilous pestilence. 4 He shall cover you with His feathers, And under His wings you shall take refuge; His truth shall be your shield and buckler. 5 You shall not be afraid of the terror by night, Nor of the arrow that flies by day, 6 Nor of the pestilence that walks in darkness, Nor of the destruction that lays waste at noonday. 7 A thousand may fall at your side, And ten thousand at your right hand; But it shall not come near you. 8 Only with your eyes shall you look, And see the reward of the*

*wicked. 9 Because you have made the Lord ,
who is my refuge, Even the Most High, your
dwelling place, 10 No evil shall befall you, Nor
shall any plague come near your dwelling; 11
For He shall give His angels charge over you,
To keep you in all your ways. 12 In their hands
they shall bear you up, Lest you dash your foot
against a stone. 13 You shall tread upon the lion
and the cobra, The young lion and the serpent
you shall trample underfoot. 14 "Because he has
set his love upon Me, therefore I will deliver
him; I will set him on high, because he has
known My name. 15 He shall call upon Me, and
I will answer him; I will be with him in trouble;
I will deliver him and honor him. 16 With long
life I will satisfy him, And show him My
salvation." NKJV*

God is my sufficiency ~

*II Corinthians 3:5 Not that we are sufficient of
ourselves to think of anything as being from
ourselves, but our sufficiency is from God, KJV*

I am more than a conqueror ~

*Romans 8:37 Yet in all these things we are
more than conquerors through Him who loved
us. NKJV*

God gives us the will and ability to do His will ~

49

> *Philippians 2:13 for it is God who works in you both to will and to do for* His *good pleasure. NKJV*

God's Acceptance of You

He has made me a beautiful creation with a purpose~

> *Ecclesiastes 3:11 He has made everything beautiful in its time. He also has planted eternity in men's hearts and minds [a divinely implanted sense of a purpose working through the ages which nothing under the sun but God alone can satisfy], yet so that men cannot find out what God has done from the beginning to the end. AMP*

He has made me a highly favored one ~

> *Ephesians 1:3-6 Blessed be the God and Father of our Lord Jesus Christ, who has blessed us with every spiritual blessing in the heavenly places in Christ, 4 just as He chose us in Him before the foundation of the world, that we should be holy and without blame before Him in love, 5 having predestined us to adoption as sons by Jesus Christ to Himself, according to the good pleasure of His will, 6 to the praise of the glory of His grace, by which He made us accepted (highly favored one) in the Beloved. NKJV*

I am God's child by His adoption ~

> *Romans 8:15-17 For you did not receive the spirit of bondage again to fear, but you received the Spirit of adoption by whom we cry out, "Abba, Father." 16 The Spirit Himself bears witness with our spirit that we are children of God, 17 and if children, then heirs — heirs of God and joint heirs with Christ, if indeed we suffer with Him, that we may also be glorified together. NKJV*

Christ has received me and adopted me as His child~

> *Romans 15:7 Therefore receive one another, just as Christ also received us, to the glory of God. NKJV*

> *Psalms 27:10 Although my father and my mother have forsaken me, yet the Lord will take me up [adopt me as His child]. AMP*

> *Psalms 94:14 For the Lord will not cast off His people, Nor will He forsake His inheritance. NKJV*

He will never leave or forsake me ~

> *Hebrews 13:5 Let your conduct be without covetousness; be content with such things as you have. For He Himself has said, "I will never leave you nor forsake you." NKJV*

> *Deuteronomy 31:6 Be strong and of good courage, do not fear nor be afraid of them; for the Lord your God, He is the One who goes with you. He will not leave you nor forsake you." NKJV*

My Victory

No weapon formed against me shall prosper ~

> *Isaiah 54:17 No weapon formed against you shall prosper, And every tongue which rises against you in judgment You shall condemn. This is the heritage of the servants of the Lord, And their righteousness is from Me," Says the Lord. NKJV*

I will live a long life ~

> *Psalms 91:16 With long life will I satisfy him and show him My salvation. NKJV*

I have the right self-talk ~

> *Psalms 103:1-5 Bless the Lord, O my soul; And all that is within me, bless His holy name! Bless the Lord, O my soul, And forget not all His benefits: Who forgives all your iniquities, Who heals all your diseases, Who redeems your life from destruction, Who crowns you with lovingkindness and tender mercies, Who satisfies your mouth with good things, So that your youth is renewed like the eagle's. NKJV*

> *Proverbs 16:24 Gracious words are like a honeycomb, sweetness to the soul and health to the body. ESV*

Starve your fears and feed your faith!

> *Luke 8:49-50 While he was still speaking, someone from the ruler's house came and said, "Your daughter is dead; do not trouble the Teacher any more." 50 But Jesus on hearing this answered him, "Do not fear; only believe, and she will be well." ESV*

What I Say Matters

> *Proverbs 18:21 Death and life are in the power of the tongue, and they who indulge in it shall eat the fruit of it [for death or life]. AMP*

> *Ezekiel 37:3-10 And he said to me, "Son of man, can these bones live?" And I answered, "O Lord God, you know." Then he said to me, "Prophesy over these bones, and say to them, O dry bones, hear the word of the Lord. Thus says the Lord God to these bones: Behold, I will cause breath to enter you, and you shall live. And I will lay sinews upon you, and will cause flesh to come upon you, and cover you with skin, and put breath in you, and you shall live, and you shall know that I am the Lord." So I prophesied as I was commanded. And as I prophesied, there was a sound, and behold, a rattling, and the bones came together, bone to its bone. And I looked, and behold, there were sinews on them, and flesh had come upon them, and skin had covered them. But there was no breath in them. Then he said to me, "Prophesy to the breath; prophesy, son of man, and say to the breath, Thus says the Lord God : Come from the four winds, O breath, and breathe on these slain, that they may live." So I prophesied as he commanded me, and the breath came into*

them, and they lived and stood on their feet, an exceedingly great army. ESV

Proverbs 18:4 The words of a [discreet and wise] man's mouth are like deep waters [plenteous and difficult to fathom], and the fountain of skillful and godly Wisdom is like a gushing stream [sparkling, fresh, pure, and life-giving]. AMP

Proverbs 10:20-21 The tongues of those who are upright and in right standing with God are as choice silver; the minds of those who are wicked and out of harmony with God are of little value. The lips of the [uncompromisingly] righteous feed and guide many, but fools die for want of understanding and heart. AMP

Proverbs 10:31 The mouths of the righteous (those harmonious with God) bring forth skillful and godly Wisdom, but the perverse tongue shall be cut down [like a barren and rotten tree]. AMP

Matthew 12:35-37 The good man from his inner good treasure flings forth good things, and the evil man out of his inner evil storehouse flings forth evil things. But I tell you, on the day of judgment men will have to give account for every idle (inoperative, nonworking) word they speak. For by your words you will be justified and acquitted, and by your words you will be condemned and sentenced. AMP

Ephesians 4:29 Let no foul or polluting language, nor evil word nor unwholesome or worthless talk [ever] come out of your mouth, but only such [speech] as is good and beneficial to the spiritual progress of others, as is fitting to the need and the occasion, that it may be a blessing and give grace (God's favor) to those who hear it. AMP

Proverbs 4:23 Guard your heart above all else, for it determines the course of your life. NLT

Colossians 4:6 Let your speech at all times be gracious (pleasant and winsome), seasoned [as it were] with salt, [so that you may never be at a loss] to know how you ought to answer anyone [who puts a question to you]. AMP

Romans 12:2 Do not be conformed to this world, but be transformed by the renewal of your mind, that by testing you may discern what is the will of God, what is good and acceptable and perfect. ESV

My Victory Is Connected To My Obedience To God's Word

Leviticus 26:14-22 "But if you will not listen to me and will not do all these commandments, if you spurn my statutes, and if your soul abhors my rules, so that you will not do all my commandments, but break my covenant, then I will do this to you: I will visit you with panic, with wasting disease and fever that consume the eyes and make the heart ache. And you shall sow your seed in vain, for your enemies shall eat it. I will set my face against you, and you shall be struck down before your enemies. Those who hate you shall rule over you, and you shall flee when none pursues you. And if in spite of this you will not listen to me, then I will discipline you again sevenfold for your sins, and I will break the pride of your power, and I will make your heavens like iron and your earth like bronze. And your strength shall be spent in vain, for your land shall not yield its increase, and the trees of the land shall not yield their fruit. "Then if you walk contrary to me and will not listen to me, I will continue striking you, sevenfold for your sins. And I will let loose the wild beasts against you, which shall bereave

> *you of your children and destroy your livestock and make you few in number, so that your roads shall be deserted. ESV*

I walk uprightly and His Words do me good ~

> *Micah 2:7 O house of Jacob, shall it be said, Is the Spirit of the Lord restricted, impatient, and shortened? Or are these [prophesied plagues] His doings? Do not My words do good to him who walks uprightly? AMP*

I will walk in the good way and heed His words and laws~

> *Jeremiah 6:16, 19 16 Thus says the Lord: "Stand in the ways and see, And ask for the old paths, where the good way is, And walk in it; Then you will find rest for your souls... 19 Hear, O earth! Behold, I will certainly bring calamity on this people — The fruit of their thoughts, Because they have not heeded My words Nor My law, but rejected it. NKJV*

> *Deuteronomy 6:17-19 You shall diligently keep the commandments of the Lord your God, His testimonies, and His statutes which He has commanded you. 18 And you shall do what is right and good in the sight of the Lord , that it may be well with you, and that you may go in and possess the good land of which the Lord swore to your fathers, 19 to cast out all your enemies from before you, as the Lord has spoken. NKJV*

Anger

I will not let the sun go down on my wrath~

> *Ephesians 4:26-27 "Be angry, and do not sin": do not let the sun go down on your wrath, 27 nor give place to the devil. NKJV*

I will be slow to get angry~

> *James 1:19-20 So then, my beloved brethren, let every man be swift to hear, slow to speak, slow to wrath; 20 for the wrath of man does not produce the righteousness of God. NKJV*

I will be slow to speak~

> *Proverbs 29:11 A fool vents all his feelings, But a wise man holds them back. NKJV*

My anger does not produce righteousness~

> *James 1:20 for the wrath of man does not produce the righteousness of God. NKJV*

I am slow to anger~

> *Proverbs 19:11 The discretion of a man makes him slow to anger, And his glory is to overlook a transgression. NKJV*

I will cease from anger~

> *Psalms 37:8 Cease from anger, and forsake wrath; Do not fret — it only causes harm. NKJV*

Outbursts of wrath are works of the flesh~

> *Galatians 5:19-20 Now the works of the flesh are evident, which are: adultery, fornication, uncleanness, lewdness, 20 idolatry, sorcery, hatred, contentions, jealousies, outbursts of wrath, selfish ambitions, dissensions, heresies, NKJV*

I will treat others as I want to be treated~

> *Luke 6:31 And just as you want men to do to you, you also do to them likewise. NKJV*

I am slow to anger and rule my spirit~

> *Proverbs 16:32 He who is slow to anger is better than the mighty, And he who rules his spirit than he who takes a city. NKJV*

I put off anger and wrath~

> *Colossians 3:8 But now you yourselves are to put off all these: anger, wrath, malice, blasphemy, filthy language out of your mouth. NKJV*

Anger rests in fools~

> *Ecclesiastes 7:9 Do not hasten in your spirit to be angry, For anger rests in the bosom of fools. NKJV*

Fear

God is my shield to protect me ~

> *Genesis 15:1 After these things the word of the Lord came to Abram in a vision, saying, "Do not be afraid, Abram. I am your shield, your exceedingly great reward." NKJV*

Because I fear the Lord He teaches me ~

> *Psalms 25:12 Who is the man that fears the Lord? Him shall He teach in the way He chooses. NKJV*

God watches over me, I will not fear ~

> *Psalms 91:5 You shall not be afraid of the terror by night, Nor of the arrow that flies by day, NKJV*

I do not need to fear bad news ~

> *Psalms 112:7 He will not be afraid of evil tidings; His heart is steadfast, trusting in the Lord. NKJV*

God is with me and strengthens and upholds me ~

> *Isaiah 41:10 Fear not, for I am with you; Be not dismayed, for I am your God. I will strengthen you, Yes, I will help you, I will uphold you with My righteous right hand.' NKJV*

God will help me ~

> *Isaiah 41:13 For I, the Lord your God, will hold your right hand, Saying to you, 'Fear not, I will help you.' NKJV*

My sleep will be sweet for God is my confidence ~

> *Proverb 3:24-26 When you lie down, you will not be afraid; Yes, you will lie down and your sleep will be sweet. 25 Do not be afraid of sudden terror, Nor of trouble from the wicked when it comes; 26 For the Lord will be your*

> *confidence, And will keep your foot from being caught. NKJV*

I have power, love and a sound mind ~

> *II Tim 1:7 For God has not given us a spirit of fear, but of power and of love and of a sound mind. NKJV*

God is my Father ~

> *Romans 8:15 For you did not receive the spirit of bondage again to fear, but you received the Spirit of adoption by whom we cry out, "Abba, Father." NKJV*

God will never leave or forsake me ~

> *Hebrews 13:5-6 Let your conduct be without covetousness; be content with such things as you have. For He Himself has said, "I will never leave you nor forsake you." 6 So we may boldly say: "The Lord is my helper; I will not fear. What can man do to me?" NKJV*

The Lord is the strength of my life ~

> *Psalms 27:1 The Lord is my light and my salvation; Whom shall I fear? The Lord is the strength of my life; Of whom shall I be afraid? NKJV*

God delivers me of all my fears ~

> *Psalms 34:4 I sought the Lord , and He heard me, And delivered me from all my fears. NKJV*

God is very present and helps me in times of trouble~

> *Psalms 46:1-3 God is our refuge and strength, A very present help in trouble. 2 Therefore we will not fear, Even though the earth be removed, And though the mountains be carried into the midst of the sea; 3 Though its waters roar and be troubled, Though the mountains shake with its swelling. NKJV*

> *Titus 3:5 he saved us, not because of works done by us in righteousness, but according to his own mercy, by the washing of regeneration and renewal of the Holy Spirit, ESV*

Whenever I go through difficulty God is with me

> *Isaiah 43:1-2 But now, thus says the Lord , who created you, O Jacob, And He who formed you, O Israel: "Fear not, for I have redeemed you; I have called you by your name; You are Mine. 2 When you pass through the waters, I will be with you; And through the rivers, they shall not overflow you. When you walk through the fire,*

> *you shall not be burned, Nor shall the flame scorch you. NKJV*

I listen to the Lord and dwell safely ~

> *Proverb 1:33 But whoever listens to me will dwell safely, And will be secure, without fear of evil." NKJV*

God is my helper ~

> *Hebrews 13:6 So we may boldly say: "The Lord is my helper; I will not fear. What can man do to me?" NKJV*

God's love drives away fear ~

> *1 John 4:18 There is no fear in love; but perfect love casts out fear, because fear involves torment. But he who fears has not been made perfect in love. NKJV*

Worry and Anxiety

I will not worry, God will take care of me ~

> *Matthew 6:25-34 "Therefore I say to you, do not worry about your life, what you will eat or what you will drink; nor about your body, what you will put on. Is not life more than food and the body more than clothing? 26 Look at the birds of the air, for they neither sow nor reap nor gather into barns; yet your heavenly*

Father feeds them. Are you not of more value than they? 27 Which of you by worrying can add one cubit to his stature? 28 "So why do you worry about clothing? Consider the lilies of the field, how they grow: they neither toil nor spin; 29 and yet I say to you that even Solomon in all his glory was not arrayed like one of these. 30 Now if God so clothes the grass of the field, which today is, and tomorrow is thrown into the oven, will He not much more clothe you, O you of little faith? 31 "Therefore do not worry, saying, 'What shall we eat?' or 'What shall we drink?' or 'What shall we wear?' 32 For after all these things the Gentiles seek. For your heavenly Father knows that you need all these things. 33 But seek first the kingdom of God and His righteousness, and all these things shall be added to you. 34 Therefore do not worry about tomorrow, for tomorrow will worry about its own things. Sufficient for the day is its own trouble. NKJV

Proverbs 4:20-27 My son, be attentive to my words; incline your ear to my sayings.21 Let them not escape from your sight; keep them within your heart.22 For they are life to those who find them, and healing to all their[a] flesh. 23 Keep your heart with all vigilance, for from it flow the springs of life. 24 Put away from you crooked speech, and put devious talk far

> *from you.25 Let your eyes look directly forward, and your gaze be straight before you. 26 Ponder[b] the path of your feet; then all your ways will be sure. 27 Do not swerve to the right or to the left; turn your foot away from evil. ESV*

I trust in my God and I have peace ~

> *Isaiah 26:3 You will keep him in perfect peace, Whose mind is stayed on You, Because he trusts in You. NKJV*

I cast my burden on the Lord and He sustains me ~

> *Psalms 55:22 Cast your burden on the Lord , And He shall sustain you; He shall never permit the righteous to be moved. NKJV*

I will make my requests known to God in prayer with a thankful heart ~

> *Philippians 4:6-7 Be anxious for nothing, but in everything by prayer and supplication, with thanksgiving, let your requests be made known to God; 7 and the peace of God, which surpasses all understanding, will guard your hearts and minds through Christ Jesus. NKJV*

Because I love God all things work out to my good ~

> *Romans 8:28 And we know that all things work together for good to those who love God, to those who are the called according to His purpose. NKJV*

I choose life and blessings for me and my offspring

> *Deuteronomy 30:19 I call heaven and earth to witness against you today, that I have set before you life and death, blessing and curse. Therefore choose life, that you and your offspring may live, ESV*

I have the peace of Jesus which is translated (health, welfare, prosperity and every kind of good) ~

> *John 14:27 Peace I leave with you, My peace I give to you; not as the world gives do I give to you. Let not your heart be troubled, neither let it be afraid. NKJV*

I will not worry about what I should say as He will teach me what to say ~

> *Luke 12:11-12 "Now when they bring you to the synagogues and magistrates and authorities, do not worry about how or what you should answer, or what you should say. 12 For the Holy Spirit will teach you in that very hour*

> *what you ought to say." NKJV*

I cast my cares on Him ~

> *I Peter 5:7 casting all your care upon Him, for He cares for you. NKJV*

I am full of courage because He has strengthened my heart ~

> *Psalms 31:24 Be of good courage, And He shall strengthen your heart, All you who hope in the Lord. NKJV*

> *Psalms 27:14 Wait on the Lord; Be of good courage, And He shall strengthen your heart; Wait, I say, on the Lord ! NKJV*

Forgiveness

God forgives my many sins ~

> *Psalms 65:3 When we were overwhelmed by sins, you forgave our transgressions. NIV*

God forgives me because He loves me ~

> *Psalms 86:50 For You, Lord, are good, and ready to forgive, And abundant in mercy to all those who call upon You. NKJV*

God makes me as clean as freshly fallen snow ~

> *Isaiah 1:18 "Come now, and let us reason together," Says the Lord, "Though your sins are like scarlet, They shall be as white as snow; Though they are red like crimson, They shall be as wool. NKJV*

God removes my impurities ~

> *Ezekiel 36:25 Then I will sprinkle clean water on you, and you shall be clean; I will cleanse you from all your filthiness and from all your idols. NKJV*

I must forgive others ~

> *Matthew 6:14-15 14 "For if you forgive men their trespasses, your heavenly Father will also forgive you. 15 But if you do not forgive men their trespasses, neither will your Father forgive your trespasses. NKJV*

I cannot keep track of how many times I have forgiven ~

> *Matthew 18:21-35 Then Peter came to Him and said, "Lord, how often shall my brother sin against me, and I forgive him? Up to seven times?" 22 Jesus said to him, "I do not say to you, up to seven times, but up to seventy times seven. 23 Therefore the kingdom of heaven is*

like a certain king who wanted to settle accounts with his servants. 24 And when he had begun to settle accounts, one was brought to him who owed him ten thousand talents. 25 But as he was not able to pay, his master commanded that he be sold, with his wife and children and all that he had, and that payment be made. 26 The servant therefore fell down before him, saying, 'Master, have patience with me, and I will pay you all.' 27 Then the master of that servant was moved with compassion, released him, and forgave him the debt. 28 "But that servant went out and found one of his fellow servants who owed him a hundred denarii; and he laid hands on him and took him by the throat, saying, 'Pay me what you owe!' 29 So his fellow servant fell down at his feet and begged him, saying, 'Have patience with me, and I will pay you all.' 30 And he would not, but went and threw him into prison till he should pay the debt. 31 So when his fellow servants saw what had been done, they were very grieved, and came and told their master all that had been done. 32 Then his master, after he had called him, said to him, 'You wicked servant! I forgave you all that debt because you begged me. 33 Should you not also have had compassion on your fellow servant, just as I had pity on you?' 34 And his master was angry, and delivered him to the torturers until he should pay all that was due to him.

> *35 "So My heavenly Father also will do to you if each of you, from his heart, does not forgive his brother his trespasses." NKJV*

I must freely forgive others as God has forgiven me ~

> *Colossians 3:13 bearing with one another, and forgiving one another, if anyone has a complaint against another; even as Christ forgave you, so you also must do. NKJV*

God will forgive my sins as I confess them ~

> *1 John 1:8-9 If we say that we have no sin, we deceive ourselves, and the truth is not in us. 9 If we confess our sins, He is faithful and just to forgive us our sins and to cleanse us from all unrighteousness. NKJV*

God has removed my sins from me ~

> *Psalms 103:12 As far as the east is from the west, So far has He removed our transgressions from us. NKJV*

God will remember my sins no more ~

> *Hebrews 8:12 For I will be merciful to their unrighteousness, and their sins and their lawless deeds I will remember no more." NKJV*

God casts my sins into the depths of the sea ~

> *Micah 7:19 He will again have compassion on us, And will subdue our iniquities. You will cast all our sins Into the depths of the sea. NKJV*

God has cast my sins behind His back~

> *Isaiah 38:17 Indeed it was for my own peace That I had great bitterness; But You have lovingly delivered my soul from the pit of corruption, For You have cast all my sins behind Your back. NKJV*

God does not remember my sins~

> *Isaiah 43:25 "I, even I, am He who blots out your transgressions for My own sake; And I will not remember your sins. NKJV*

Because I am in Christ, all things are new~

> *2 Corinthians 5:17 Therefore, if anyone is in Christ, he is a new creation; old things have passed away; behold, all things have become new. NKJV*

Thoughts

My thoughts must be guarded as sin starts with a thought ~

> *Matthew 5:27-30 "You have heard that it was said to those of old, 'You shall not commit adultery.' 28 But I say to you that whoever*

> *looks at a woman to lust for her has already committed adultery with her in his heart. 29 If your right eye causes you to sin, pluck it out and cast it from you; for it is more profitable for you that one of your members perish, than for your whole body to be cast into hell. 30 And if your right hand causes you to sin, cut it off and cast it from you; for it is more profitable for you that one of your members perish, than for your whole body to be cast into hell. NKJV*

My mind is being transformed and renewed ~

> *Romans 12:2 And do not be conformed to this world, but be transformed by the renewing of your mind, that you may prove what is that good and acceptable and perfect will of God. NKJV*

My fellowship with God helps me make decisions by spiritual wisdom ~

> *1 Corinthians 2:6-16 However, we speak wisdom among those who are mature, yet not the wisdom of this age, nor of the rulers of this age, who are coming to nothing. 7 But we speak the wisdom of God in a mystery, the hidden wisdom which God ordained before the ages for our glory, 8 which none of the rulers of this age knew; for had they known, they would not have crucified the Lord of glory. 9 But as it is written: "Eye has not seen, nor ear heard, Nor*

have entered into the heart of man The things which God has prepared for those who love Him." 10 But God has revealed them to us through His Spirit. For the Spirit searches all things, yes, the deep things of God. 11 For what man knows the things of a man except the spirit of the man which is in him? Even so no one knows the things of God except the Spirit of God. 12 Now we have received, not the spirit of the world, but the Spirit who is from God, that we might know the things that have been freely given to us by God. 13 These things we also speak, not in words which man's wisdom teaches but which the Holy Spirit teaches, comparing spiritual things with spiritual. 14 But the natural man does not receive the things of the Spirit of God, for they are foolishness to him; nor can he know them, because they are spiritually discerned. 15 But he who is spiritual judges all things, yet he himself is rightly judged by no one. 16 For "who has known the mind of the Lord that he may instruct Him?" But we have the mind of Christ. NKJV

I bring every thought into captivity ~

2 Corinthians 10:3-6 For though we walk in the flesh, we do not war according to the flesh. 4 For the weapons of our warfare are not carnal but mighty in God for pulling down strongholds, 5 casting down arguments and every high thing that exalts itself against the knowledge of God, bringing every thought into captivity to the obedience of Christ, 6 and being ready to punish all disobedience when your obedience is fulfilled. NKJV

I should please God with my thoughts ~

Philippians 4:8 Finally, brethren, whatever things are true, whatever things are noble, whatever things are just, whatever things are pure, whatever things are lovely, whatever things are of good report, if there is any virtue and if there is anything praiseworthy — meditate on these things. NKJV

I must guard my thoughts ~

Proverbs 4:23 Keep your heart with all diligence, For out of it spring the issues of life. NKJV

Sin wars against my mind ~

Romans 7:23 But I see another law in my members, warring against the law of my mind, and bringing me into captivity to the law of sin which is in my members. NKJV

I refuse to be double-minded ~

James 1:8 he is a double-minded man, unstable in all his ways. NKJV

Faith

I can do all things ~

> *Philippians 4:13 I can do all things through Christ who strengthens me. NKJV*

I believe despite what I see ~

> *Hebrews 11:1-2 Now faith is the substance of things hoped for, the evidence of things not seen. 2 For by it the elders obtained a good testimony. NKJV*

> *II Corinthians 5:7 For we walk by faith, not by sight. NKJV*

I do not doubt what God has said ~

> *James 1:5-6 If any of you lacks wisdom, let him ask of God, who gives to all liberally and without reproach, and it will be given to him. 6 But let him ask in faith, with no doubting, for he who doubts is like a wave of the sea driven and tossed by the wind. NKJV*

I abound in faith with thanksgiving ~

> *Colossians 2:6-7 As you therefore have received Christ Jesus the Lord, so walk in Him, 7 rooted and built up in Him and established in the faith, as you have been taught, abounding in it with*

> *thanksgiving. NKJV*

My faith is in Jesus ~

> *Galatians 2:20 I have been crucified with Christ; it is no longer I who live, but Christ lives in me; and the life which I now live in the flesh I live by faith in the Son of God, who loved me and gave Himself for me. NKJV*

I speak to my mountain ~

> *Mark 11:22-24 So Jesus answered and said to them, "Have faith in God. 23 For assuredly, I say to you, whoever says to this mountain, 'Be removed and be cast into the sea,' and does not doubt in his heart, but believes that those things he says will be done, he will have whatever he says. 24 Therefore I say to you, whatever things you ask when you pray, believe that you receive them, and you will have them. NKJV*

I read the Word to boost my faith ~

> *Romans 10:17 So then faith comes by hearing, and hearing by the word of God. NKJV*

I feed my faith and starve my doubts ~

> *Matthew 17:20-21 So Jesus said to them, "Because of your unbelief; for assuredly, I say to you, if you have faith as a mustard seed, you will say to this mountain, 'Move from here to*

> *there,' and it will move; and nothing will be impossible for you. 21 However, this kind does not go out except by prayer and fasting." NKJV*

My faith is more precious than gold ~

> *I Peter 1:7 that the genuineness of your faith, being much more precious than gold that perishes, though it is tested by fire, may be found to praise, honor, and glory at the revelation of Jesus Christ, NKJV*

My faith overcomes the world ~

> *I John 5:4 For whatever is born of God overcomes the world. And this is the victory that has overcome the world — our faith. NKJV*

I have faith and I speak to all obstacles in my way ~

> *Luke 17:5-6 And the apostles said to the Lord, "Increase our faith." 6 So the Lord said, "If you have faith as a mustard seed, you can say to this mulberry tree, 'Be pulled up by the roots and be planted in the sea,' and it would obey you. NKJV*

I quench all the fiery darts of the enemy with my shield of faith ~

> *Ephesians 6:16 above all, taking the shield of faith with which you will be able to quench all the fiery darts of the wicked one. NKJV*

Rejection

The Lord delivers me of all rejection ~

> *Psalms 34:17-20 The righteous cry out, and the Lord hears, And delivers them out of all their troubles. 18 The Lord is near to those who have a broken heart, And saves such as have a contrite spirit. 19 Many are the afflictions of the righteous, But the Lord delivers him out of them all. 20 He guards all his bones; Not one of them is broken. NKJV*

Though I am rejected by man I am precious to God ~

> *1 Peter 2:4 Coming to Him as to a living stone, rejected indeed by men, but chosen by God and precious, NKJV*

Jesus was rejected and overcame rejection on my behalf ~

> *John 15:18 "If the world hates you, you know that it hated Me before it hated you. NKJV*

> *Isaiah 53:3 He is despised and rejected by men,*
> *A Man of sorrows and acquainted with grief.*
> *And we hid, as it were, our faces from Him; He*
> *was despised, and we did not esteem Him.*
> *NKJV*

> *Psalms 118:22 The stone which the builders*
> *rejected Has become the chief cornerstone.*
> *NKJV*

I am sober and vigilant ~

> *1 Peter 5:8 Be sober, be vigilant; because your*
> *adversary the devil walks about like a roaring*
> *lion, seeking whom he may devour. NKJV*

I cast my care on Him ~

> *1 Peter 5:7 casting all your care upon Him, for*
> *He cares for you. NKJV*

Rejection is a doctrine of demons ~

> *1 Timothy 4:1 Now the Spirit expressly says*
> *that in latter times some will depart from the*
> *faith, giving heed to deceiving spirits and*
> *doctrines of demons, NKJV*

God has not rejected me ~

> *Romans 8:15 For you did not receive the spirit of bondage again to fear, but you received the Spirit of adoption by whom we cry out, "Abba, Father." NKJV*

One last resource on rejection that I want to include is a transcript of a portion of a message by T.D. Jakes. I have taken it verbatim from a video on YouTube.

There are people who can walk away from you, and hear me when I tell you this, when people can walk away from you, let them walk! When people can walk away from you let them walk! I can sit down now-- I've preached! I can sit down! I don't need to make an altar call or nothing. I don't have to whoop. I don't have to make you shout. I have just preached right now! When people can walk away from you. Let them walk. I don't want you to try to talk another person into staying with you, loving you, calling you, caring about you, coming to see you, staying in touch with you. I mean, hang up the phone. When people can walk away from you, let them walk! I don't care how wonderful they are. I don't care how attracted you are to them. I don't care what they did for you 20 years ago. I don't care what the situation is. When people can walk away from you, let them walk-- because your destiny is not tied to the person who left! You don't hear me—you don't want me this morning, you better leave me alone! You better run out of here. Don't let my voice fool you. There's nothing wrong with my head! Your destiny is never tied to anybody that left. The Bible says that they came out from us, that it might be made manifest that they were not of us. For had they been of us, no doubt they would have continued with us. People leave you, because they're not joined to you. And if they're not joined to you, you can get superglue and you can't make them stay. Let em go. And it doesn't mean that Orpah was a bad person. It just means that Orpah's part in the story is over and you've got to know when people's part in your story is over... So that you don't keep trying to raise the dead. You've got to know when it's dead. David, when your boy is dead wash your face and have another baby! You've got to know that it's over! Oh my God, my God, my God. Look at somebody and say nothing just happens. If they walked away, it's no accident. If they left, it's no accident. If you tried to make it work and it wouldn't work, it's no accident, accept it as the will of God. Clap your hands, wash your face, do your dance, keep going. Let me tell you something, I've got the gift of goodbye. I mean I've got the gift of goodbye. It's the 10th spiritual gift, I believe in goodbye. It's not that I'm hateful, it's that I'm faithful. And I know that whatever God needs for me to have, He will give it to me. And if it takes too much sweat, I don't need it. Stop begging people to stay. Let them go![5]

I included the quote above by T.D. Jakes because so many of us tend to get focused on what someone has or hasn't done, especially as it relates to our being or felling rejected. We need to come to the place where we realize we do not need to remain a victim of others, it is our choice! May you find your freedom from rejection!

"Thank you for reading this book! We have covered a lot of ground here, and I am confident that the information provided will help you in your journey to healing and wholeness. I would ask you to do two things: Apply what you have learned NOW (not tomorrow), and gain your healing and wholeness! Help other potential readers that are in the same situation that you were in before reading this book. Please take a minute to submit a Review on the Amazon website here http://www.amazon.com/Freedom-Endometriosis-Everyone-Ought-Bethesda/dp/1484086058/

**See our other books and CDs on Amazon.com[6]

---

[5] http://www.youtube.com/watch?v=Pketb6gxR3w

[6] http://www.amazon.com/Dr.-Robert-B.-Campbell/e/B00DRGNZLU/ref=ntt_athr_dp_pel_1

<u>"Freedom From Endometriosis"</u>

Some reviews from Amazon

~ After 10.5 years of marriage, and being given no hope from the doctors for 'natural conception', I decided to dedicate a few months to the principals in Dr. Robert Campbell's book. I found much truth in his insight into endometriosis.
My husband and I had gone through years of surgeries and procedures after finding out in 2010 that I had upper-stage 3 endometriosis. The medical community could do nothing for me at that time except try and help me conceive to 'kill off' the endometriosis (which is hormone fed) to which we suffered the loss of 4 babies early term. We battled through polyps, fibroids, common cysts and endometrium cyst along with excruciating pain emotionally and physically. Years later, we purchased Dr. Campbell's book at a conference and dedicated a few months to its principals. I'm pleased to say that this February (2014), we found out we were naturally pregnant (with less than 1% chance, according to the doctors) for the first time in our lives with our miracle baby. And now we are almost through our first trimester and feeling amazing. Alongside the physical healing, I found I was more free emotionally because of the book. (BTW, the baby arrived!)

"Freedom From Migraines"

Some reviews from Amazon

~ *I was having a rough week in terms of taking on rejection and false guilt. Wednesday that week was a particular rough day and I knew it, but it was like I was so caught up in it, I couldn't drag myself out of it. The next afternoon rolled around and I got a pre-migraine aura. They usually last for about 45 minutes and then the nauseating headache begins and I'm in bed the rest of the day and vomiting. BUT, I spent that 45 minutes repenting of my awful thoughts and going through your freedom from migraines book. And guess what??? NO HEADACHE!!! :)*

~*This book has changed my life! It never crossed my mind before that our headaches could be caused by guilt.*

~*I'm truly grateful for Dr. Campbell's approach with Migraines. I've had several clients suffer from them and Dr. Campbell's knowledge has assisted me & them tremendously. I must read for anyone who has or knows anyone that suffers from Migraines. What a gift to have Dr. Campbell's expertise right on my kindle.*

"Freedom From Acid Reflux"

Some reviews from Amazon

~ *As I was reading through this book I was thinking about the people who I would like to give a copy to* ease their suffering! The text contained a list of foods and beverages that exacerbate the episodes as well as the causes. There is a common denominator with this condition and many illnesses that people today struggle with which is totally overlooked by the medical community, the mind-emotion-body connection. The body was designed for these three components to be in harmony and when one of these components is out of balance, it causes the other two to become unbalanced as well, creating an impaired immune system. The author presents a viable solution to this dilemma without costing you valuable resources. I find it refreshing that by following the process he outlines suffering can be alleviated and people can be free to live a normal life style in moderation.

<u>"Freedom From High Blood Pressure"</u>

Some reviews from Amazon

~ As a physician, I am always looking at alternative medicine options. This is a good read and am interested in testing its application.

~this is a great book I am a high blood pressure patient...i most definitely recommend reading this wonderful book...thank you

<u>"Freedom From Asthma"</u>

Some reviews from Amazon

~ This book truly hit home for me. I was diagnosed

with asthma at the age of 30 (53 now). Friends would ask "are you allergic to your husband"? I laughed it off however, deep down I knew there was something more to it. I have been working on this disease ever since. After reading such a powerful book my Asthma has improved (still more false-guilt issues I'm working through)

Thank You Dr. Campbell for giving me an "outsider looking in" approach.

~ After years of treating the symptoms of asthma with my children, we are finally understanding the roots causes. That is something that no doctor has been able to give us adequate answers about. We have been told told by the medical community to stop looking for the cause of asthma and just worry about the symptoms. After reading Freedom from Asthma we are able to approach asthma very differently. Understanding that the root causes of asthma are spiritual has changed our lives. I am so thankful to have these tools as we battle asthma in our family. Finally, someone is addressing the the root causes of asthma and how to combat them.

"Freedom From Eczema"

Some reviews from Amazon

~ Eczema is a skin condition that effects 9-30% of the U.S. population according to the National Institute of Arthritis and Musculoskeletal and Skin Diseases (see [...] The cause of eczema is unknown by the medical *community but through the power of Scripture, healing is possible. Dr. Robert Campbell's "Freedom from Eczema" offers practical ways on overcoming this condition. I've seen first hand individuals impacted by the teachings in this book where they've received freedom from eczema and continue to walk in freedom from it. You have all to gain and nothing to lose! I highly encourage you to read and apply these principles and see how the power of prayer and Scripture can transform your life into a life of victory!*

"Freedom From Allergies"

Some reviews from Amazon

~ My family battled with allergies for many years. The information presented in this book set us FREE! Whatever your physical battle is, you will find freedom by applying the truths in this book! Dr. Robert Campbell has a heart to help others find freedom!

"Freedom From Acne"

Some reviews from Amazon

~ When I was a teenager, my Dr. recommended that I take an antibiotic long term (for about 6 months I was on it) and it just messed me up internally. I had to suffer side effects, and had to re-balance my system from now having too much candida with the antibiotics. I've tried many topical remedies as well. But what works the best, is getting to the source of

your acne, and solving that. Here is a solution that will decrease stress and anxiety in your life - a major contributor to acne!

~ I struggled with acne throughout my teenage years and into my 20s. I wish I would have had this resource doing those days. So much struggle with not only the acne itself could have been avoided but all the self-esteem issues that went along with it! Thank God for doctors and medicine but this is vital information for those interested in complete healing and freedom from this common nemesis!

<u>"Freedom From Diabetes Type I & II"</u>

Some reviews from Amazon

~ I found this book very informative! My husband has been dealing with type 2 diabetes for 15 years. I appreciate the depth to which the author discusses both types of diabetes, making comparisons and highlighting the latest research with its implications. The information which I found alarming is the risk of heart disease and stroke are 2-4 times greater for those people who have diabetes in addition to the fact they are more likely to get severe cases of the flu. I was surprised to read that both types are connected to either a reaction of the immune system or malfunction of the immune system which are triggered by environmental factors. I am grateful to this author who looks at other approaches to treating disease than the traditional protocol which only *treats the symptoms and not the roots. If you apply the knowledge outlined in this book it will give you the power to take control of what is ultimately a life threatening disease.*

<u>"Freedom Form Strokes"</u>

Some reviews from Amazon

~ I regret that I didn't have this information prior to December 26, 2012 because that is when my mother passed away from stroke due to atrial fibrillation. i would highly recommend for every person to read this book so you will have no regrets. It is educational and could some day save your life or the life of someone you love.

<u>"Freedom Form Breast Cancer"</u>

Some reviews from Amazon

~ I was diagnosed with breast cancer this week and this book has helped me get through some rough patches. So many passages from the bible that were exactly what I need.

<u>"Freedom Form Psoriasis"</u>

Some reviews from Amazon

~ This book is so full of insights that you freedom in so many areas of your life - not just psoriasis. Illnesses have root causes that doctors don't discuss. Doctors treat symptoms, but don't help us explore why our bodies are stressed and get sick to begin with. This

book answers that and brings freedom from anxiety, fear, stress, and so much more which is the real cause to us getting sick. ~

Through these principles and walking in authority through Christ, I've been healed of many things such as scoliosis (medically proven to be gone). I was healed of scoliosis immediately after dealing with deep rejection in my life and the moment I prayed, it was instantly gone. I have X-rays and witnesses. God still heals and He very much loves you. Be blessed. ~Teresa

<u>"Freedom From Depression"</u>

The Bible is the best resource for not just spiritual needs but for our physical and emotional needs as well. Dr. Campbell nails the truth about depression, how and why it works and what God says it takes to get out from under its grip. Depression is becoming an epidemic in our nation. If you have been struggling with depression and/or anxiety this teaching will help you greatly. I also recommend this book to anyone who is close to someone struggling with depression. As you gain insights into this disorder you will be more effective in assisting those suffering from depression to succeed. I like how Dr. Campbell brings the Bible to life with authoritative scripture teaching that is effective and powerful. I received a copy of this book about 2 months ago and I continue to use this book and reference it as often as I need to. During the last three years I have been on various medications, made dietary changes, tried various vitamins and herbal remedies and so far I have gained more relief from the teachings in "Freedom from Depression" than any of these other treatments. ~Ralph

I believe Everyone needs to hear this teaching....It is very practical but yet powerful.....as the bible says we MUST renew our mind...The chemical changes that happen when we are stressed or afraid, etc. help contribute to many ill effects...Dr Bob Campbell goes into great depths of teaching on this subject....It makes perfect sense to the natural man......Dr Bob Campbell even explains how low level discouragement is a form of depression....
.I actually had a 7 week class at my church with this teaching and wrote out an outline to study........You will be surprised at what you will learn from this teaching.....
Thank you for this understanding.....this will give many hopeless a new found hope, without drugs that cover, shock treatments that cause memory loss and expensive coping sessions.....we need to get to the root and have God heal us from here on out by the power of His word with the renewing of our mind Thank you, I am stronger because of it and I have hope again...~ Cathy Catania

You can also purchase our books and other resources at

www.booksandgiftstogo.org and use promo code

2OOFF code at checkout for a 20% discount!

<u>Authority of the Believe Pool Of Bethesda Healing Series I MP3s</u>

<u>Authority of the Believe Pool Of Bethesda Healing Series II MP3s</u>

<u>Authority of the Believe Pool Of Bethesda Healing SeriesIII MP3s</u>

<u>Authority of the Believer Pt. I, II and III Healing MP3s</u>

<u>The Authority Of The Believer Vol 1-3 USB Card with 8 Videos</u>

Email me at <u>ignitedministriesinternational@gmail.com</u>

with questions or testimonies.

**See our book "Breaking Free From Rejection". Email me at poolofbethesdaschoolofhealing@gmail.com

---

[i] Don Colbert M.D.. Deadly Emotions: Understand the Mind-Body-Spirit Connection That Can Heal or Destroy You (Kindle Locations 269-270). Kindle Edition.

[ii] Don Colbert M.D.. Deadly Emotions: Understand the Mind-Body-Spirit Connection That Can Heal or Destroy You (Kindle Locations 283-284). Kindle Edition.

[iii] http://www.nimh.nih.gov/health/publications/anxiety-disorders/complete-

index.shtml

iv http://www.wnd.com/2013/04/americans-snapping-by-the-millions/print/
v http://www.fearofstuff.com/featured/10-famous-people-who-have-phobias/

vi http://www.webmd.com/balance/stress-management/features/10-fixable-stress-related-health-problems
vii http://www.merriam-webster.com/dictionary/fear
viii http://en.wikipedia.org/wiki/Fear
ix http://www.helpguide.org/mental/phobia_symptoms_types_treatment.htm

x http://www.sermonillustrations.com/a-z/f/fear.htm
xi http://m.kidshealth.org/teen/your_mind/mental_health/phobias.html
xii http://www.sermonillustrations.com/a-z/f/fear.htm
xiii Don Colbert M.D.. Deadly Emotions: Understand the Mind-Body-Spirit Connection That Can Heal or Destroy You (Kindle Locations 245-249). Kindle Edition.
xiv http://www.sermonillustrations.com/a-z/f/fear.htm
xv http://biblicalcounselinginsights.com/attitudes-and-behaviors/fear-vs-faith/
xvi
http://books.google.com/books?id=GJAnaY4KCPMC&pg=PA121&lpg=PA121&dq=Janez+Rus+wartime&source=bl&ots=BG2yi6W_3x&sig=pmt_0bVsjYl1F3wR5S0E-rf15gQ&hl=en&sa=X&ei=_NeFUeHIIsXy0QHX04CoCQ&ved=0CDAQ6AEwAA#v=onepage&q=Janez%20Rus%20wartime&f=false
xvii (from Greek-English Lexicon Based on Semantic Domain. Copyright © 1988 United Bible Societies, New York. Used by permission.)
xviii http://www.opposite-word.com/o/of%20sound%20mind
xix (Biblesoft's New Exhaustive Strong's Numbers and Concordance with Expanded Greek-Hebrew Dictionary. Copyright © 1994, 2003, 2006 Biblesoft, Inc. and International Bible Translators, Inc.)

xx (from Greek-English Lexicon Based on Semantic Domain. Copyright © 1988 United Bible Societies, New York. Used by permission.)

xxi Complete Word Study Bible
xxii (from The Complete Word Study Dictionary: New Testament © 1992 by AMG International, Inc. Revised Edition, 1993)

xxiii (from The Complete Word Study Dictionary: New Testament © 1992 by AMG International, Inc. Revised Edition, 1993)

[xxiv] (from The Complete Word Study Dictionary: New Testament © 1992 by AMG International, Inc. Revised Edition, 1993)

[xxv] (from The Complete Word Study Dictionary: New Testament © 1992 by AMG International, Inc. Revised Edition, 1993)

[xxvi] Zechariah 4:6

[xxvii] (from The Complete Word Study Dictionary: New Testament © 1992 by AMG International, Inc. Revised Edition, 1993)

[xxviii] (from The Complete Word Study Dictionary: New Testament © 1992 by AMG International, Inc. Revised Edition, 1993)

[xxix] Numbers 14:37 NKJV

[xxx] http://phobialist.com/class.html

[xxxi] http://m.kidshealth.org/teen/your_mind/mental_health/phobias.html

[xxxii] The preceding excerpt is taken from Chapter 12 of Colon & Rectal Cancer: A Comprehensive Guide for Patients & Families by Lorraine Johnston, copyright 2000 by O'Reilly & Associates, Inc.